1-WEEK FULL-BODY DETOX DIET

Revitalize your body in 7-days: Discover the ultimate full-body detox diet for weight loss, energy, vitality and optimal health with simple step and delicious recipes

Odesa Mulan

Table of Contents

CHAPTER ONE 6
- Understanding the Importance of Detoxification for Overall Health 6
- What is Detoxification? 6
- The Importance of Detoxification for Overall Health 7
- Methods of Detoxification 9
- Conclusion 11

CHAPTER TWO 12
- Preparing Mentally and Physically for a 1-Week Detox Journey 12
- Understanding the Purpose of Detox 12
- Setting Clear Goals 13
- Creating a Supportive Environment 13
- Educating Yourself 13
- Gradual Transition 14
- Hydration 14
- Mindfulness and Stress Reduction 14
- Meal Planning and Preparation 15
- Seeking Professional Guidance 15
- Maintaining a Positive Mindset 15
- Conclusion 16

CHAPTER THREE 17
Setting Clear Goals and Intentions for Your Detox Week........ 17
Reflecting on Your Why 17
SMART Goals 18
Examples of Detox Goals....................................... 19
Visualizing Success 20
Tracking Progress and Celebrating Success..................... 21
Conclusion 21

CHAPTER FOUR 22
Day 1: Jumpstarting Your Detox with Fresh Juices and Smoothies 22
Benefits of Fresh Juices and Smoothies 22
Creating Detox-Friendly Juices and Smoothies 24
Sample Juices and Smoothies for Day 1........................ 26
Conclusion 27

CHAPTER FIVE 28
Day 2: Eliminating Toxins with Whole Foods and Herbal Teas 28
The Role of Whole Foods in Detoxification..................... 28
Incorporating Whole Foods into Your Detox Day 30
The Benefits of Herbal Teas for Detoxification 32
Conclusion 34

CHAPTER SIX 35

Day 3: Supporting Digestive Health with Fiber-Rich Foods and Herbal Supplements 35

The Importance of Digestive Health in Detoxification 36

Fiber-Rich Foods for Digestive Health..................................36

Herbal Supplements for Digestive Support............................38

Sample Day 3 Menu..39

Conclusion 41

CHAPTER SEVEN...42

Day 4: Rejuvenating Your Body with Detoxifying Herbs and Spices 42

The Benefits of Detoxifying Herbs and Spices........................42

Incorporating Detoxifying Herbs and Spices into Your Day 4 Detox Plan 44

CHAPTER EIGHT..48

Day 5: Hydrating and Cleansing Your System with Herbal Infusions 48

The Benefits of Herbal Infusions 48

Incorporating Herbal Infusions into Your Day 5 Detox Plan 50

Conclusion 52

CHAPTER NINE 54

Day 6: Mind-Body Practices for Detoxification and Stress Reduction 54

The Importance of Mind-Body Practices in Detoxification 54

Mind-Body Practices for Day 6 Detox 55

Creating Your Day 6 Mind-Body Detox Routine 58

Conclusion 59

CHAPTER TEN 60

Day 7: Reflecting on Your Detox Week and Creating a Post-Detox Plan 60

BONUS 66

SOME HOLISTIC APPROACHES TO KNOW 66

THE END 86

COPYRIGHT © 2023

All rights reserved. No part of this publication may be reproduced, distributed, or transmitted in any form or by any means, including photocopying, recording, or other electronic or mechanical methods, without the prior written permission of the publisher, except in the case of brief quotations embodied in critical reviews and certain other noncommercial uses permitted by copyright law.

CHAPTER ONE

Understanding the Importance of Detoxification for Overall Health

Detoxification, often shortened to detox, is a process that involves eliminating toxins and harmful substances from the body. While the body has its natural detoxification mechanisms, environmental pollutants, unhealthy diets, stress, and other factors can overwhelm these systems, leading to a buildup of toxins. Detoxification practices aim to support and enhance the body's natural detox processes, promoting overall health and well-being.

What is Detoxification?

Detoxification is the body's process of removing harmful substances, known as toxins, through various organs such as the liver, kidneys, skin, lungs, and digestive system. These toxins can come from both external sources, such as environmental pollutants, pesticides, and heavy metals, as well as internal sources like metabolic waste products and harmful by-products of cellular processes.

The liver plays a central role in detoxification, as it metabolizes and neutralizes toxins before they are eliminated from the body. The kidneys filter toxins from the blood and excrete them in the urine, while the digestive system removes waste and toxins through bowel movements. Additionally, the skin eliminates toxins through sweat, and the lungs expel toxins through respiration.

The Importance of Detoxification for Overall Health

Detoxification is crucial for maintaining optimal health and well-being for several reasons:

1. **Removal of Toxins:** Over time, the body accumulates toxins from various sources, which can impair cellular function, contribute to inflammation, and increase the risk of chronic diseases such as cancer, cardiovascular disease, and neurological disorders. Detoxification helps eliminate these toxins, reducing the burden on organs and tissues and promoting overall health.

2. **Enhanced Nutrient Absorption:** When toxins accumulate in the body, they can interfere with nutrient absorption and utilization. By eliminating toxins through detoxification, the body can better absorb essential nutrients from food, supporting overall health and vitality.

3. **Improved Energy Levels:** Toxins and metabolic waste products can sap energy and contribute to fatigue and sluggishness. Detoxification helps rejuvenate the body's

energy systems, leading to increased vitality, mental clarity, and overall well-being.

4. **Supports Weight Management:** Toxins stored in fat cells can interfere with metabolic processes and contribute to weight gain and obesity. By eliminating toxins through detoxification, individuals may experience improved metabolism, better weight management, and enhanced body composition.

5. **Boosts Immune Function:** A healthy immune system is essential for defending the body against pathogens and maintaining overall health. Detoxification supports immune function by reducing the burden of toxins and promoting optimal functioning of immune cells and tissues.

6. **Promotes Healthy Aging:** As we age, the body's detoxification capacity may decline, leading to an accumulation of toxins and an increased risk of age-related diseases. Detoxification practices can help slow the aging process by supporting the body's natural detox mechanisms and reducing oxidative stress and inflammation.

Methods of Detoxification

There are various methods of detoxification, ranging from dietary changes and lifestyle modifications to specialized detox programs and therapies. Some common approaches to detoxification include:

1. **Healthy Diet:** Eating a balanced diet rich in fruits, vegetables, whole grains, lean proteins, and healthy fats provides essential nutrients and supports the body's natural detox processes. Avoiding processed foods, sugar, alcohol, caffeine, and artificial additives can reduce the intake of toxins and support detoxification.

2. **Hydration:** Drinking an adequate amount of water is essential for flushing toxins from the body and supporting kidney function. Staying hydrated helps maintain optimal detoxification pathways and promotes overall health and well-being.

3. **Exercise:** Regular physical activity stimulates circulation, promotes sweating, and supports the lymphatic system, all of which aid in detoxification. Incorporating activities such as brisk walking, cycling, swimming, and yoga can enhance the body's natural detox processes.

4. **Sauna Therapy:** Saunas induce sweating, which helps eliminate toxins through the skin. Sweating in a sauna can promote detoxification, improve circulation, and support overall health and well-being.

5. **Supplements:** Certain supplements and herbs, such as milk thistle, dandelion root, turmeric, and glutathione, can support liver function and enhance detoxification pathways. However, it's essential to consult with a healthcare

professional before taking any supplements, as they may interact with medications or have adverse effects.

6. **Colon Cleansing:** Colon cleansing involves flushing out the colon with water or other liquids to remove accumulated waste and toxins. While some people believe that colon cleansing can improve detoxification and promote weight loss, there is limited scientific evidence to support its effectiveness and safety.

7. **Fasting:** Fasting involves abstaining from food for a specific period, allowing the body to rest and detoxify. Intermittent fasting, juice fasting, and water fasting are some common fasting protocols used for detoxification purposes. However, fasting should be done under the guidance of a healthcare professional, as it may not be suitable for everyone and can have potential risks.

8. **Mind-Body Practices:** Stress management techniques such as meditation, deep breathing, and yoga can support detoxification by reducing stress hormones and promoting relaxation. Stress reduction is essential for overall health and well-being and can enhance the body's natural detox processes.

Conclusion

Detoxification is a vital process for maintaining overall health and well-being. By supporting the body's natural detox mechanisms through dietary changes, lifestyle modifications, and specialized detox therapies, individuals can reduce the burden of toxins, improve energy levels, boost immune function, and promote healthy aging. However, it's essential to approach detoxification safely and under the guidance of a healthcare professional to ensure effectiveness and minimize potential risks. By incorporating detoxification practices into a healthy lifestyle, individuals can optimize their health and vitality for years to come.

CHAPTER TWO

Preparing Mentally and Physically for a 1-Week Detox Journey

Embarking on a one-week detox journey can be a transformative experience for both the body and mind. However, proper preparation is essential to ensure a successful and rewarding detoxification process. This preparation involves not only making physical adjustments to your diet and lifestyle but also cultivating the right mindset to support your journey towards improved health and well-being.

Understanding the Purpose of Detox

Before diving into a one-week detox journey, it's crucial to understand the purpose behind it. Detoxification aims to eliminate toxins from the body, support vital organs such as the liver and kidneys, and promote overall health and well-being. By removing toxins accumulated from environmental pollutants, processed foods, alcohol, caffeine, and other sources, detoxification can rejuvenate the body's natural detox processes and restore balance.

Setting Clear Goals

Setting clear and realistic goals is essential for a successful detox journey. Whether your goals include weight loss, increased energy levels, improved digestion, or simply feeling better overall, having a clear understanding of what you hope to achieve can help you stay focused and motivated throughout the process. Write down your goals and revisit them regularly to stay on track and monitor your progress.

Creating a Supportive Environment

Creating a supportive environment is key to ensuring a successful detox journey. Surround yourself with positive influences, whether it's supportive friends and family members, online communities, or healthcare professionals who can offer guidance and encouragement. Communicate your intentions with those close to you and enlist their support in your detox journey.

Educating Yourself

Educating yourself about the principles of detoxification, healthy eating, and lifestyle habits is crucial for making informed choices during your detox journey. Research reputable sources, consult with healthcare professionals, and familiarize yourself with detox-friendly foods, recipes, and meal plans. Understanding how different foods and lifestyle factors impact your body can empower you to make healthier choices and maximize the benefits of detoxification.

Gradual Transition

Rather than diving into a detox program abruptly, consider making gradual transitions to prepare your body and mind for the changes ahead. Start by gradually reducing your intake of processed foods, sugar, caffeine, and alcohol in the days leading up to your detox. Focus on incorporating more whole, nutrient-dense foods such as fruits, vegetables, whole grains, lean proteins, and healthy fats into your diet to nourish your body and support detoxification.

Hydration

Proper hydration is essential for supporting detoxification and overall health. Start increasing your water intake in the days leading up to your detox journey to ensure you're adequately hydrated. Consider incorporating hydrating foods such as cucumbers, watermelon, and leafy greens into your diet to boost hydration levels and support the body's natural detox processes.

Mindfulness and Stress Reduction

Practicing mindfulness and stress reduction techniques can help prepare you mentally and emotionally for your detox journey. Incorporate activities such as meditation, deep breathing exercises, yoga, or journaling into your daily routine to promote relaxation, reduce stress hormones, and cultivate a positive mindset. Remember that detoxification is not just about cleansing the body but also nurturing the mind and spirit.

Meal Planning and Preparation

Meal planning and preparation are essential for staying on track during your detox journey. Take time to plan out your meals and snacks for the week, ensuring they're balanced, nourishing, and aligned with your detox goals. Consider batch cooking and prepping meals in advance to save time and make healthy eating more convenient. Stock up on detox-friendly ingredients and remove any tempting or unhealthy foods from your home to minimize temptation.

Seeking Professional Guidance

If you're new to detoxification or have specific health concerns, consider seeking guidance from a healthcare professional or nutritionist before starting your detox journey. They can provide personalized recommendations, address any potential risks or contraindications, and offer support and guidance throughout the process. Your healthcare provider can also help you determine the most appropriate detox approach based on your individual needs and goals.

Maintaining a Positive Mindset

Maintaining a positive mindset is essential for navigating challenges and setbacks during your detox journey. Embrace the process as an opportunity for growth, self-discovery, and positive change. Celebrate your successes, no matter how small, and practice self-compassion and forgiveness if you veer off course. Remember that detoxification is a journey, not a destination, and focus on progress rather than perfection.

Conclusion

Preparing mentally and physically for a one-week detox journey requires thoughtful planning, education, and commitment. By setting clear goals, creating a supportive environment, gradually transitioning to a detox-friendly diet, practicing mindfulness and stress reduction, and seeking professional guidance when needed, you can maximize the benefits of detoxification and embark on a journey towards improved health and well-being. Remember to approach the process with an open mind and a positive attitude, embracing the opportunity for growth and transformation.

CHAPTER THREE

Setting Clear Goals and Intentions for Your Detox Week

Embarking on a detox week can be a powerful step towards rejuvenating your body and revitalizing your health. Setting clear goals and intentions is essential for guiding your journey and maximizing the benefits of detoxification. By defining what you hope to achieve and why, you can stay focused, motivated, and aligned with your vision for a healthier lifestyle.

Reflecting on Your Why

Before setting specific goals for your detox week, take some time to reflect on your reasons for undertaking this journey. Ask yourself why you feel compelled to detoxify your body and what you hope to gain from the experience. Your motivations might include improving your energy levels, supporting your immune system, kickstarting weight loss, reducing inflammation, enhancing mental clarity, or simply feeling better overall. Understanding your underlying motivations will help you set meaningful and relevant goals for your detox week.

SMART Goals

When setting goals for your detox week, it's helpful to follow the SMART criteria, which stands for Specific, Measurable, Achievable, Relevant, and Time-bound. SMART goals provide a clear framework for goal-setting and increase the likelihood of success. Here's how you can apply the SMART criteria to your detox goals:

1. **Specific:** Clearly define what you want to accomplish during your detox week. Instead of setting vague goals like "improve my health," be specific about the outcomes you're aiming for, such as "increase energy levels," "reduce bloating," or "eliminate sugar cravings."

2. **Measurable:** Determine how you will measure progress towards your goals. This could involve tracking specific metrics such as weight, body measurements, energy levels, mood, or adherence to your detox plan. Measurable goals allow you to assess your progress objectively and make adjustments as needed.

3. **Achievable:** Ensure that your goals are realistic and attainable within the timeframe of your detox week. Consider your current health status, lifestyle habits, and any potential challenges or limitations. Setting achievable goals increases your confidence and motivation to succeed.

4. **Relevant:** Your detox goals should align with your overall health priorities and reasons for undertaking the detox week. Focus on goals that are relevant to your specific needs and aspirations, whether they relate to physical health, mental well-being, emotional balance, or lifestyle habits.

5. **Time-bound:** Set a specific timeframe for achieving your goals, in this case, the duration of your detox week. Having a deadline creates a sense of urgency and accountability, motivating you to take action and stay committed to your goals throughout the week.

Examples of Detox Goals

Here are some examples of SMART goals you might set for your detox week:

1. **Increase Energy Levels:** "During my detox week, I will prioritize getting at least 8 hours of sleep each night and incorporate daily exercise to boost my energy levels and reduce fatigue."

2. **Eliminate Sugar Cravings:** "For the duration of my detox week, I will eliminate all refined sugars and processed foods from my diet and focus on consuming whole, nutrient-dense foods to curb sugar cravings."

3. **Support Digestive Health:** "Throughout my detox week, I will incorporate fiber-rich foods such as fruits, vegetables, and whole grains into my meals to support digestive health and alleviate bloating and discomfort."

4. **Hydration:** "I will drink at least 8 glasses of water each day during my detox week to stay hydrated and support the body's natural detoxification processes."

5. **Mindfulness and Stress Reduction:** "During my detox week, I will practice daily meditation and deep breathing exercises to reduce stress levels, promote relaxation, and enhance mental clarity and focus."

6. **Meal Planning and Preparation:** "I will dedicate time each weekend to plan and prepare detox-friendly meals and snacks for the upcoming week, ensuring that I have nourishing options readily available to support my detox goals."

Visualizing Success

Visualization is a powerful tool for manifesting your goals and intentions. Take time each day to visualize yourself achieving your detox goals and experiencing the benefits of a healthier, revitalized body and mind. Imagine how you will feel, look, and function once you've successfully completed your detox week. Visualizing success reinforces your commitment to your goals and motivates you to take consistent action towards achieving them.

Tracking Progress and Celebrating Success

Throughout your detox week, track your progress towards your goals and celebrate small victories along the way. Keep a journal to record your daily experiences, observations, and any changes you notice in your body and mind. Celebrate milestones, no matter how small, and acknowledge the progress you've made towards improving your health and well-being. By tracking your progress and celebrating success, you'll stay motivated and inspired to continue prioritizing your health beyond the detox week.

Conclusion

Setting clear goals and intentions is essential for a successful detox week. By reflecting on your why, setting SMART goals, visualizing success, tracking progress, and celebrating achievements, you can stay focused, motivated, and aligned with your vision for a healthier lifestyle. Remember that detoxification is not just about cleansing the body but also nurturing the mind and spirit. Approach your detox week with positivity, intention, and a commitment to your well-being, and you'll emerge feeling refreshed, revitalized, and empowered to continue prioritizing your health in the long term.

CHAPTER FOUR

Day 1: Jumpstarting Your Detox with Fresh Juices and Smoothies

As you embark on your detox journey, Day 1 sets the tone for the rest of the week. Jumpstarting your detox with fresh juices and smoothies can provide your body with essential nutrients, hydrate your cells, and kickstart your metabolism. By fueling your body with nutrient-dense ingredients, you'll support its natural detoxification processes and lay the foundation for a successful week of cleansing and rejuvenation.

Benefits of Fresh Juices and Smoothies

Fresh juices and smoothies offer a convenient and delicious way to flood your body with vitamins, minerals, antioxidants, and phytonutrients. Here are some key benefits of incorporating fresh juices and smoothies into your detox day:

1. **Hydration:** Both juices and smoothies provide hydration to your body, which is essential for supporting detoxification and maintaining overall health. Hydration helps flush out toxins, supports cellular function, and keeps your skin glowing and radiant.

2. **Nutrient Absorption:** Fresh juices and smoothies deliver a concentrated dose of nutrients that are easily absorbed by your body. By consuming fruits and vegetables in liquid form,

you bypass the need for digestion, allowing your body to quickly access and utilize the nutrients for optimal health and vitality.

3. **Alkalizing Properties:** Many detox-friendly ingredients, such as leafy greens, cucumbers, and celery, have alkalizing properties that help balance the body's pH levels. Alkaline-forming foods promote detoxification, reduce inflammation, and support overall well-being.

4. **Digestive Support:** Certain ingredients commonly used in juices and smoothies, such as ginger, mint, and probiotic-rich foods like yogurt or kefir, can support digestion and soothe the gastrointestinal tract. These ingredients help alleviate bloating, gas, and digestive discomfort, promoting a healthy gut environment.

5. **Energy Boost:** Fresh juices and smoothies provide a natural source of energy to fuel your body and mind throughout the day. By nourishing your cells with nutrient-rich ingredients, you'll experience sustained energy levels without the crashes associated with caffeine or sugar.

Creating Detox-Friendly Juices and Smoothies

When preparing your juices and smoothies for Day 1 of your detox, focus on using whole, organic ingredients that are rich in vitamins, minerals, and antioxidants. Aim to include a variety of fruits, vegetables, leafy greens, and superfoods to maximize the nutritional benefits. Here are some detox-friendly ingredients to consider:

1. **Leafy Greens:** Spinach, kale, Swiss chard, and collard greens are excellent sources of vitamins A, C, and K, as well as minerals like iron, calcium, and magnesium. Add a handful of leafy greens to your juices and smoothies for a nutrient boost.

2. **Citrus Fruits:** Oranges, lemons, limes, and grapefruits are high in vitamin C, which supports immune function and collagen production. Citrus fruits also add a refreshing flavor to your juices and smoothies.

3. **Berries:** Blueberries, strawberries, raspberries, and blackberries are rich in antioxidants called anthocyanins, which help combat oxidative stress and inflammation. Berries add sweetness and vibrant color to your detox beverages.

4. **Cucumbers:** Cucumbers are hydrating and alkalizing, making them an ideal ingredient for detox juices and smoothies. They're also low in calories and high in vitamins K and B, as well as minerals like potassium and magnesium.

5. **Celery:** Celery is a natural diuretic that helps flush out excess fluids and toxins from the body. It's also rich in electrolytes,

such as potassium and sodium, which support hydration and cellular function.

6. **Ginger:** Ginger has anti-inflammatory and digestive properties that can help soothe the stomach and alleviate nausea. Add a small piece of fresh ginger root to your juices and smoothies for a zesty kick.

7. **Turmeric:** Turmeric contains curcumin, a potent antioxidant with anti-inflammatory properties. Adding a pinch of turmeric powder or fresh turmeric root to your detox beverages can help reduce inflammation and support detoxification.

8. **Leafy Herbs:** Fresh herbs like mint, parsley, cilantro, and basil add flavor and nutritional benefits to your juices and smoothies. Mint helps soothe digestion, while parsley and cilantro support detoxification by binding to heavy metals and facilitating their excretion.

Sample Juices and Smoothies for Day 1

Here are some simple yet delicious recipes to jumpstart your detox on Day 1:

1. **Green Detox Juice:**
    - Ingredients: Spinach, cucumber, celery, green apple, lemon, ginger

- Directions: Juice all ingredients in a blender or juicer. Stir well and enjoy immediately.

2. **Berry Detox Smoothie:**

    - Ingredients: Mixed berries (blueberries, strawberries, raspberries), spinach, banana, almond milk, chia seeds

    - Directions: Blend all ingredients until smooth and creamy. Pour into a glass and garnish with a sprinkle of chia seeds.

3. **Citrus Immunity Booster:**

    - Ingredients: Oranges, grapefruit, lemon, ginger, turmeric, honey (optional)

    - Directions: Juice the citrus fruits, ginger, and turmeric. Stir in honey if desired. Serve chilled over ice.

4. **Tropical Green Smoothie:**

    - Ingredients: Pineapple, mango, spinach, coconut water, Greek yogurt (optional)

    - Directions: Blend all ingredients until smooth. Add Greek yogurt for extra creaminess, if desired.

5. **Detoxifying Green Tea Smoothie:**

    - Ingredients: Green tea (brewed and cooled), kale, cucumber, pear, lemon juice, honey (optional)

- Directions: Brew green tea and let it cool. Blend with kale, cucumber, pear, lemon juice, and honey until smooth.

Conclusion

Day 1 of your detox journey sets the stage for a week of rejuvenation and renewal. By jumpstarting your detox with fresh juices and smoothies packed with nutrient-dense ingredients, you'll nourish your body, support its natural detoxification processes, and lay the foundation for a healthier lifestyle. Experiment with different combinations of fruits, vegetables, leafy greens, and superfoods to discover your favorite detox beverages. Remember to stay hydrated, listen to your body's cues, and enjoy the delicious flavors and benefits of your detox creations. Cheers to a revitalizing Day 1 and a week of vibrant health ahead!

CHAPTER FIVE

Day 2: Eliminating Toxins with Whole Foods and Herbal Teas

On Day 2 of your detox journey, you'll continue to support your body's natural detoxification processes by focusing on whole foods and herbal teas. By eliminating processed foods, sugar, caffeine, and other potential toxins from your diet and incorporating nutrient-rich foods and detoxifying herbs, you'll nourish your body from the inside out and facilitate the elimination of harmful substances. Additionally, herbal teas provide hydration and therapeutic benefits that support detoxification and promote overall well-being.

The Role of Whole Foods in Detoxification

Whole foods are foods that are minimally processed and as close to their natural state as possible. They provide essential nutrients, including vitamins, minerals, antioxidants, and fiber, that support overall health and well-being. When it comes to detoxification, whole foods play a crucial role in nourishing the body and supporting its natural detox processes. Here's how whole foods contribute to detoxification:

1. **Nutrient Density:** Whole foods are rich in vitamins, minerals, and antioxidants that support cellular function, repair, and regeneration. By consuming a variety of nutrient-dense

foods, you provide your body with the essential nutrients it needs to fuel detoxification pathways and maintain optimal health.

2. **Fiber Content:** Whole foods such as fruits, vegetables, whole grains, legumes, and nuts are rich in dietary fiber, which supports digestive health and regular bowel movements. Fiber helps sweep toxins and waste products out of the digestive tract, preventing them from being reabsorbed into the body.

3. **Hydration:** Many whole foods, such as fruits and vegetables, have high water content, which contributes to hydration and supports the body's natural detox processes. Proper hydration is essential for flushing out toxins, supporting kidney function, and maintaining overall health.

4. **Antioxidant Activity:** Whole foods contain antioxidants, such as vitamins A, C, and E, as well as phytonutrients like flavonoids and polyphenols, which help neutralize free radicals and reduce oxidative stress. Antioxidants protect cells from damage caused by toxins and support detoxification at the cellular level.

5. **Liver Support:** Certain whole foods, including cruciferous vegetables like broccoli, cauliflower, and Brussels sprouts, as well as sulfur-rich foods like garlic and onions, support liver function and enhance detoxification pathways. These foods

contain compounds that stimulate enzyme activity and promote the elimination of toxins from the body.

Incorporating Whole Foods into Your Detox Day

On Day 2 of your detox journey, focus on incorporating a variety of whole foods into your meals and snacks. Choose organic, seasonal, and locally sourced ingredients whenever possible to minimize exposure to pesticides, herbicides, and other harmful chemicals. Here are some detox-friendly whole foods to include in your Day 2 menu:

1. **Leafy Greens:** Spinach, kale, Swiss chard, collard greens, and arugula are nutrient powerhouses rich in vitamins, minerals, and antioxidants. Incorporate leafy greens into salads, smoothies, stir-fries, soups, and wraps for a nutritional boost.

2. **Colorful Vegetables:** Fill your plate with a rainbow of vegetables, including bell peppers, carrots, tomatoes, cucumbers, zucchini, eggplant, and beets. These vegetables provide a variety of vitamins, minerals, and phytonutrients that support detoxification and overall health.

3. **Whole Grains:** Choose whole grains such as quinoa, brown rice, oats, barley, and buckwheat over refined grains to maximize fiber and nutrient content. Whole grains provide

sustained energy, support digestive health, and help stabilize blood sugar levels.

4. **Lean Proteins:** Opt for lean sources of protein such as poultry, fish, tofu, tempeh, legumes, and lentils. Protein is essential for tissue repair and muscle maintenance and can help keep you feeling satisfied and energized throughout the day.

5. **Healthy Fats:** Include sources of healthy fats such as avocados, nuts, seeds, and olive oil in your meals and snacks. Healthy fats provide essential fatty acids that support brain function, hormone production, and cellular health.

6. **Detoxifying Herbs and Spices:** Incorporate detoxifying herbs and spices such as turmeric, ginger, garlic, cilantro, parsley, and dandelion greens into your meals. These herbs and spices have anti-inflammatory, antioxidant, and liver-supportive properties that aid in detoxification.

The Benefits of Herbal Teas for Detoxification

In addition to whole foods, herbal teas are an excellent way to support detoxification and promote overall well-being. Herbal teas are made from a variety of dried herbs, flowers, roots, and leaves, each with its unique therapeutic properties. Here are some benefits of incorporating herbal teas into your detox day:

1. **Hydration:** Herbal teas provide hydration without the added sugars, caffeine, or artificial additives found in many other beverages. Staying hydrated is essential for supporting detoxification, promoting digestion, and maintaining overall health.

2. **Liver Support:** Certain herbs, such as dandelion root, milk thistle, burdock root, and chicory root, support liver function and enhance detoxification pathways. These herbs contain compounds that stimulate bile production, promote liver detoxification, and support the elimination of toxins from the body.

3. **Digestive Health:** Many herbs used in herbal teas, such as peppermint, ginger, fennel, and chamomile, have digestive benefits that help soothe the stomach, alleviate bloating, and support overall digestive health. These herbs promote the flow of digestive juices, reduce inflammation, and calm gastrointestinal discomfort.

4. **Antioxidant Activity:** Herbal teas are rich in antioxidants, including polyphenols, flavonoids, and catechins, which help protect cells from oxidative damage caused by toxins and free radicals. Antioxidants support detoxification at the cellular level and promote overall health and longevity.

5. **Relaxation and Stress Reduction:** Many herbal teas have calming and relaxing properties that help reduce stress,

promote relaxation, and support mental well-being. Ingredients such as chamomile, lavender, lemon balm, and passionflower can help soothe the nervous system and promote restful sleep.

Sample Whole Foods and Herbal Teas for Day 2

Here are some ideas for incorporating whole foods and herbal teas into your Day 2 detox menu:

Breakfast:

- Green smoothie made with spinach, banana, pineapple, almond milk, and chia seeds
- Herbal tea blend of peppermint, ginger, and lemon balm for digestion support

Lunch:

- Quinoa salad with mixed vegetables (bell peppers, cucumber, cherry tomatoes, avocado), chickpeas, and lemon-tahini dressing
- Herbal tea infusion of dandelion root, burdock root, and licorice for liver support

Snack:

- Sliced cucumber and carrot sticks with hummus
- Herbal tea blend of chamomile and lavender for relaxation

Dinner:

- Baked salmon with roasted Brussels sprouts and sweet potatoes
- Herbal tea infusion of ginger, turmeric, and lemon for anti-inflammatory support

Evening Snack:

- Greek yogurt with mixed berries and a drizzle of honey
- Herbal tea blend of chamomile, lemon balm, and passionflower for relaxation and sleep support

Conclusion

Day 2 of your detox journey focuses on eliminating toxins with whole foods and herbal teas. By incorporating a variety of nutrient-rich whole foods into your meals and snacks and enjoying detoxifying herbal teas throughout the day, you'll support your body's natural detoxification processes and promote overall health and well-being. Experiment with different flavors, ingredients, and herbal tea blends to discover what works best for you. Stay hydrated, listen to your body's cues, and savor the delicious flavors and benefits of your detox-friendly meals and beverages. Cheers to a nourishing and rejuvenating Day 2 of your detox journey!

CHAPTER SIX

Day 3: Supporting Digestive Health with Fiber-Rich Foods and Herbal Supplements

On Day 3 of your detox journey, you'll focus on supporting digestive health with fiber-rich foods and herbal supplements. A healthy digestive system is essential for effective detoxification, as it plays a central role in eliminating toxins and waste products from the body. By incorporating fiber-rich foods and herbal supplements that promote digestive function, you'll help keep your digestive system running smoothly and optimize the detoxification process.

The Importance of Digestive Health in Detoxification

Digestive health is closely linked to detoxification, as the digestive system is responsible for processing and eliminating toxins and waste products from the body. When the digestive system is functioning optimally, it can efficiently break down food, absorb nutrients, and eliminate waste through bowel movements. However, factors such as poor diet, stress, lack of exercise, and certain medications can disrupt digestive function and impair detoxification pathways. Supporting digestive health during your detox journey is essential for ensuring the effective elimination of toxins and promoting overall well-being.

Fiber-Rich Foods for Digestive Health

Fiber is an essential nutrient that plays a crucial role in digestive health. It adds bulk to stool, promotes regular bowel movements, and helps prevent constipation and digestive discomfort. By incorporating fiber-rich foods into your diet, you can support digestive function and enhance the detoxification process. Here are some examples of fiber-rich foods to include in your Day 3 menu:

1. **Whole Grains:** Choose whole grains such as oats, quinoa, brown rice, barley, and bulgur for their high fiber content. These grains provide both soluble and insoluble fiber, which help regulate bowel movements and promote digestive health.

2. **Legumes:** Beans, lentils, chickpeas, and other legumes are excellent sources of fiber, protein, and complex carbohydrates. Adding legumes to your meals can increase satiety, support blood sugar control, and promote digestive regularity.

3. **Fruits:** Incorporate a variety of fruits into your diet, including apples, pears, berries, oranges, and kiwi. These fruits are rich in soluble fiber, vitamins, and antioxidants that support digestive health and overall well-being.

4. **Vegetables:** Load up on a colorful array of vegetables such as leafy greens, broccoli, cauliflower, carrots, bell peppers, and

Brussels sprouts. Vegetables are packed with fiber, vitamins, minerals, and phytonutrients that promote digestive function and detoxification.

5. **Seeds and Nuts:** Include seeds and nuts such as chia seeds, flaxseeds, hemp seeds, almonds, and walnuts in your diet for a boost of fiber and healthy fats. These foods provide essential nutrients that support digestive health and overall nutrition.

Herbal Supplements for Digestive Support

In addition to fiber-rich foods, herbal supplements can provide targeted support for digestive health during your detox journey. Certain herbs and botanicals have been traditionally used to promote digestion, relieve bloating and gas, and support the liver and gallbladder. Here are some herbal supplements to consider incorporating into your Day 3 detox regimen:

1. **Psyllium Husk:** Psyllium husk is a soluble fiber derived from the seeds of the Plantago ovata plant. It acts as a bulk-forming laxative, absorbing water in the digestive tract and promoting regular bowel movements. Adding psyllium husk to water or smoothies can help relieve constipation and support digestive health.

2. **Aloe Vera:** Aloe vera has soothing and anti-inflammatory properties that can help calm gastrointestinal irritation and promote healing of the digestive tract. Drinking aloe vera

juice or taking aloe vera supplements can support digestive health and relieve symptoms of digestive discomfort.

3. **Digestive Enzymes:** Digestive enzymes are proteins that help break down food into smaller, more easily digestible molecules. Supplementing with digestive enzymes can support the digestion of fats, carbohydrates, and proteins, reducing bloating, gas, and indigestion.

4. **Probiotics:** Probiotics are beneficial bacteria that colonize the gut and support digestive health. They help maintain a healthy balance of gut microbiota, improve digestion, boost immune function, and reduce inflammation. Consider taking a probiotic supplement or consuming probiotic-rich foods such as yogurt, kefir, sauerkraut, and kimchi.

5. **Digestive Bitters:** Herbal bitters such as gentian, dandelion, and artichoke stimulate the production of digestive juices and enzymes, enhancing digestion and nutrient absorption. Taking digestive bitters before meals can support digestion, relieve bloating, and promote liver and gallbladder function.

Sample Day 3 Menu

Here's a sample menu for Day 3 of your detox journey, featuring fiber-rich foods and herbal supplements for digestive support:

Breakfast:

- Overnight oats made with rolled oats, chia seeds, almond milk, sliced bananas, and a drizzle of honey
- Herbal tea blend of ginger, peppermint, and fennel for digestion support

Lunch:

- Quinoa salad with mixed greens, cherry tomatoes, cucumber, bell peppers, chickpeas, and a lemon-tahini dressing
- Aloe vera juice or aloe vera supplement for digestive soothing

Snack:

- Carrot and celery sticks with hummus
- Herbal tea infusion of chamomile, ginger, and licorice for relaxation and digestion support

Dinner:

- Baked salmon with roasted Brussels sprouts, sweet potatoes, and steamed broccoli
- Psyllium husk mixed with water or added to a smoothie for fiber support

Evening Snack:

- Greek yogurt topped with mixed berries, almonds, and a sprinkle of ground flaxseeds

- Probiotic supplement or probiotic-rich yogurt for gut health support

Conclusion

Day 3 of your detox journey focuses on supporting digestive health with fiber-rich foods and herbal supplements. By incorporating whole grains, legumes, fruits, vegetables, seeds, and nuts into your meals and snacks, you'll provide your body with essential nutrients and fiber to support digestive function and promote detoxification. Additionally, herbal supplements such as psyllium husk, aloe vera, digestive enzymes, probiotics, and digestive bitters can provide targeted support for digestive health and overall well-being. Experiment with different foods and supplements to find what works best for you, and remember to listen to your body's cues and stay hydrated throughout the day. Cheers to a day of nourishing and supporting your digestive system on your detox journey!

CHAPTER SEVEN

Day 4: Rejuvenating Your Body with Detoxifying Herbs and Spices

As you continue your detox journey, Day 4 presents an opportunity to rejuvenate your body with the power of detoxifying herbs and spices. These natural ingredients are rich in antioxidants, anti-inflammatory compounds, and phytonutrients that support the body's detoxification processes, promote cellular health, and boost overall well-being. By incorporating a variety of detoxifying herbs and spices into your meals and beverages, you'll nourish your body from the inside out and enhance the benefits of your detox regimen.

The Benefits of Detoxifying Herbs and Spices

Detoxifying herbs and spices have been used for centuries in traditional medicine systems for their therapeutic properties. These natural ingredients contain a wide range of bioactive compounds that support detoxification, reduce inflammation, protect against oxidative stress, and promote overall health. Here are some key benefits of incorporating detoxifying herbs and spices into your Day 4 detox plan:

1. **Liver Support:** Many detoxifying herbs and spices, such as turmeric, ginger, dandelion root, and milk thistle, support liver function and enhance detoxification pathways. These

herbs stimulate bile production, promote liver detoxification enzymes, and help eliminate toxins from the body.

2. **Anti-Inflammatory Properties:** Chronic inflammation is linked to various health issues, including digestive disorders, autoimmune conditions, and cardiovascular disease. Detoxifying herbs and spices such as turmeric, ginger, cinnamon, and cloves have potent anti-inflammatory properties that help reduce inflammation and promote tissue repair.

3. **Antioxidant Activity:** Antioxidants are compounds that neutralize free radicals and protect cells from oxidative damage. Many detoxifying herbs and spices, including cloves, cinnamon, oregano, and rosemary, are rich in antioxidants that help combat oxidative stress and promote cellular health.

4. **Digestive Support:** Certain herbs and spices, such as ginger, fennel, peppermint, and coriander, support digestive health by promoting the flow of digestive juices, reducing bloating and gas, and soothing gastrointestinal discomfort. These herbs aid in the digestion of food and support the elimination of waste products from the body.

5. **Metabolic Support:** Some detoxifying herbs and spices, such as cayenne pepper, black pepper, and green tea, have thermogenic properties that boost metabolism and support

weight management. These herbs increase energy expenditure, enhance fat oxidation, and may aid in detoxification by promoting the breakdown and elimination of toxins.

Incorporating Detoxifying Herbs and Spices into Your Day 4 Detox Plan

On Day 4 of your detox journey, focus on incorporating a variety of detoxifying herbs and spices into your meals, snacks, and beverages. These natural ingredients can be used in both savory and sweet dishes to add flavor, aroma, and therapeutic benefits. Here are some ways to incorporate detoxifying herbs and spices into your Day 4 detox plan:

1. **Turmeric:** Add ground turmeric to your morning smoothie, oatmeal, or yogurt bowl for its anti-inflammatory and liver-supportive properties. You can also make turmeric tea by steeping fresh turmeric root or turmeric powder in hot water with lemon and honey.

2. **Ginger:** Brew a cup of ginger tea by steeping fresh ginger slices in hot water or adding ginger powder to herbal tea blends. Use ginger in stir-fries, soups, salad dressings, and smoothies for its digestive and anti-inflammatory benefits.

3. **Cinnamon:** Sprinkle ground cinnamon on top of oatmeal, yogurt, or fruit salads for a delicious and warming flavor. Add

cinnamon to your morning coffee or tea for an antioxidant boost, or incorporate it into baked goods, smoothies, and desserts.

4. **Garlic:** Use fresh garlic in savory dishes such as stir-fries, soups, sauces, and marinades for its immune-boosting and detoxifying properties. Garlic contains sulfur compounds that support liver detoxification and promote cardiovascular health.

5. **Cayenne Pepper:** Add a pinch of cayenne pepper to savory dishes, salad dressings, and sauces for a spicy kick and metabolic boost. Cayenne pepper contains capsaicin, a compound that increases thermogenesis and promotes fat burning.

6. **Dandelion Root:** Brew a cup of dandelion root tea by steeping dried dandelion root in hot water for 10-15 minutes. Dandelion root tea supports liver detoxification, promotes bile flow, and aids in the elimination of toxins from the body.

7. **Cilantro:** Use fresh cilantro leaves as a garnish for salads, soups, tacos, and curries to add flavor and detoxifying benefits. Cilantro contains compounds that bind to heavy metals and facilitate their excretion from the body.

8. **Peppermint:** Enjoy a cup of peppermint tea after meals to support digestion and relieve bloating and gas. Peppermint tea has a refreshing flavor and cooling effect that helps soothe the digestive tract and promote relaxation.

Sample Day 4 Menu

Here's a sample menu for Day 4 of your detox journey, featuring detoxifying herbs and spices:

Breakfast:

- Golden turmeric smoothie made with almond milk, banana, mango, turmeric, ginger, black pepper, and a pinch of cinnamon

- Herbal tea blend of ginger, lemon, and honey for digestion support

Lunch:

- Quinoa Buddha bowl with roasted vegetables (sweet potatoes, Brussels sprouts, cauliflower), chickpeas, avocado, and a tahini-turmeric dressing

- Dandelion root tea with lemon for liver support

Snack:

- Apple slices with almond butter and a sprinkle of cinnamon

- Peppermint tea for digestion support and freshness

Dinner:

- Baked salmon with garlic-herb quinoa and steamed broccoli
- Mixed green salad with cucumber, cherry tomatoes, radishes, and a cilantro-lime dressing
- Herbal tea blend of chamomile, fennel, and licorice for relaxation and digestion support

Evening Snack:

- Greek yogurt parfait with mixed berries, granola, and a drizzle of honey
- Herbal tea infusion of chamomile, ginger, and cinnamon for relaxation and digestive support

Conclusion

Day 4 of your detox journey focuses on rejuvenating your body with the power of detoxifying herbs and spices. By incorporating a variety of herbs and spices into your meals, snacks, and beverages, you'll support liver function, reduce inflammation, promote digestion, and enhance the detoxification process. Experiment with different flavors and combinations to create delicious and nourishing meals that support your health and well-being. Cheers to a day of rejuvenation and vitality on your detox journey!

CHAPTER EIGHT

Day 5: Hydrating and Cleansing Your System with Herbal Infusions

As you reach Day 5 of your detox journey, it's time to focus on hydrating and cleansing your system with the power of herbal infusions. Herbal infusions are beverages made by steeping dried herbs, flowers, roots, or leaves in hot water, allowing their beneficial compounds to be extracted. These natural brews are rich in antioxidants, vitamins, minerals, and phytonutrients that support hydration, promote detoxification, and boost overall well-being. By incorporating a variety of herbal infusions into your Day 5 detox plan, you'll nourish your body, soothe your senses, and enhance the benefits of your detox regimen.

The Benefits of Herbal Infusions

Herbal infusions offer a multitude of health benefits, making them an excellent choice for hydrating and cleansing your system during a detox. Here are some key benefits of incorporating herbal infusions into your Day 5 detox plan:

1. **Hydration:** Staying properly hydrated is essential for supporting detoxification, maintaining cellular function, and promoting overall health. Herbal infusions provide a delicious and refreshing way to increase your fluid intake and keep your body hydrated throughout the day.

2. **Detoxification:** Many herbs used in herbal infusions, such as dandelion root, burdock root, nettle, and cleavers, support liver and kidney function and enhance the body's natural detoxification processes. These herbs help eliminate toxins, waste products, and excess fluids from the body, promoting cleansing and rejuvenation.

3. **Digestive Support:** Certain herbs, such as peppermint, ginger, fennel, and chamomile, have digestive benefits that help soothe the stomach, alleviate bloating and gas, and support overall digestive health. Herbal infusions can aid digestion, promote regular bowel movements, and relieve gastrointestinal discomfort.

4. **Antioxidant Protection:** Herbal infusions are rich in antioxidants, including polyphenols, flavonoids, and catechins, that help neutralize free radicals and protect cells from oxidative damage. Antioxidants support cellular health, reduce inflammation, and promote longevity.

5. **Relaxation and Stress Reduction:** Many herbs used in herbal infusions, such as chamomile, lavender, lemon balm, and passionflower, have calming and relaxing properties that help reduce stress, promote relaxation, and support mental well-being. Enjoying a cup of herbal tea can help you unwind and de-stress after a busy day.

Incorporating Herbal Infusions into Your Day 5 Detox Plan

On Day 5 of your detox journey, focus on incorporating a variety of herbal infusions into your daily routine to support hydration, cleansing, and overall well-being. Herbal infusions can be enjoyed hot or cold, depending on your preference, and can be customized with different herbs and flavors to suit your taste. Here are some ways to incorporate herbal infusions into your Day 5 detox plan:

1. **Morning Hydration:** Start your day with a cup of warm lemon water to hydrate your body, stimulate digestion, and alkalize your system. Squeeze the juice of half a lemon into a mug of warm water and enjoy first thing in the morning.

2. **Throughout the Day:** Sip on a variety of herbal infusions throughout the day to stay hydrated and support detoxification. Choose from a wide range of herbs and flavors, including detoxifying herbs like dandelion root, burdock root, nettle, and cleavers, as well as soothing herbs like chamomile, peppermint, ginger, and lemon balm.

3. **After Meals:** Enjoy a cup of herbal tea after meals to aid digestion and promote relaxation. Herbal teas such as ginger, fennel, peppermint, and chamomile can help soothe the stomach, relieve bloating and gas, and support overall digestive health.

4. **Before Bed:** Wind down in the evening with a calming herbal infusion to promote relaxation and prepare your body for restful sleep. Chamomile, lavender, lemon balm, and passionflower are excellent choices for bedtime teas that help reduce stress and promote a sense of calm.

Sample Day 5 Herbal Infusions

Here are some simple and delicious herbal infusion recipes to incorporate into your Day 5 detox plan:

1. **Dandelion Root Detox Tea:**

    - Ingredients: Dried dandelion root

    - Directions: Steep 1 teaspoon of dried dandelion root in a cup of hot water for 10-15 minutes. Strain and enjoy as is or sweeten with honey or stevia if desired.

2. **Ginger-Lemon Digestive Tea:**

    - Ingredients: Fresh ginger slices, lemon slices

    - Directions: Place a few slices of fresh ginger and lemon in a mug, and pour hot water over them. Let steep for 5-10 minutes, then sip and enjoy.

3. **Peppermint-Nettle Cleansing Infusion:**

    - Ingredients: Dried peppermint leaves, dried nettle leaves

- Directions: Combine equal parts dried peppermint leaves and nettle leaves in a teapot or infuser. Pour hot water over the herbs and let steep for 5-7 minutes. Strain and enjoy.

4. **Chamomile-Lavender Relaxation Tea:**

    - Ingredients: Dried chamomile flowers, dried lavender buds
    - Directions: Mix together dried chamomile flowers and lavender buds in a tea infuser. Steep in hot water for 5-7 minutes, then strain and relax with a soothing cup of tea.

5. **Turmeric-Ginger Immunity Booster:**

    - Ingredients: Ground turmeric, fresh ginger slices
    - Directions: Add a teaspoon of ground turmeric and a few slices of fresh ginger to a mug. Pour hot water over the herbs and let steep for 5-10 minutes. Stir well and enjoy.

Conclusion

Day 5 of your detox journey focuses on hydrating and cleansing your system with the power of herbal infusions. By incorporating a variety of detoxifying herbs and spices into your daily routine, you'll support hydration, promote detoxification, aid digestion, and enhance overall well-being. Experiment with different herbal infusions to discover your favorite flavors and combinations, and enjoy the soothing and therapeutic benefits of herbal tea throughout the day. Cheers to a day of hydration, cleansing, and rejuvenation on your detox journey!

CHAPTER NINE

Day 6: Mind-Body Practices for Detoxification and Stress Reduction

As you approach the final stretch of your detox journey, Day 6 is an opportune time to incorporate mind-body practices that support both detoxification and stress reduction. The mind and body are intricately connected, and practices that promote relaxation, mindfulness, and emotional well-being can enhance the effectiveness of your detox regimen. By integrating mind-body practices into your Day 6 routine, you'll not only support the body's natural detox processes but also cultivate a sense of calm, balance, and inner peace.

The Importance of Mind-Body Practices in Detoxification

Mind-body practices encompass a wide range of techniques and disciplines that focus on the connection between the mind, body, and spirit. These practices have been shown to have profound effects on physical health, mental well-being, and emotional balance. When it comes to detoxification, incorporating mind-body practices can:

1. **Reduce Stress:** Chronic stress can have detrimental effects on health and well-being, contributing to inflammation, hormonal imbalances, and impaired detoxification. Mind-

body practices such as meditation, deep breathing, and yoga can help reduce stress levels, promote relaxation, and support the body's natural detox processes.

2. **Enhance Detoxification:** Stress reduction techniques stimulate the relaxation response, which has been shown to enhance detoxification pathways in the body. By calming the nervous system and reducing stress hormones like cortisol, mind-body practices create an optimal environment for detoxification to occur.

3. **Promote Emotional Healing:** Detoxification is not just about cleansing the physical body; it also involves releasing emotional toxins and traumas stored in the mind and spirit. Mind-body practices such as mindfulness meditation, journaling, and expressive arts therapy can help process and release emotional blockages, promoting inner healing and transformation.

4. **Support Overall Well-Being:** By nurturing the mind-body connection, mind-body practices promote holistic health and well-being. They help cultivate self-awareness, self-compassion, and resilience, empowering individuals to make healthier choices and live more fulfilling lives.

Mind-Body Practices for Day 6 Detox

On Day 6 of your detox journey, dedicate time to incorporating a variety of mind-body practices that promote detoxification and stress reduction. These practices can be done individually or combined to create a personalized self-care routine that nourishes your mind, body, and spirit. Here are some effective mind-body practices to consider:

1. **Meditation:** Take time to practice meditation, focusing on deep breathing, mindfulness, and relaxation. Find a quiet and comfortable space, close your eyes, and bring your awareness to the present moment. Allow thoughts to come and go without judgment, and cultivate a sense of inner peace and stillness.

2. **Deep Breathing Exercises:** Practice deep breathing exercises to activate the body's relaxation response and reduce stress. Try diaphragmatic breathing, also known as belly breathing, by inhaling deeply through your nose, filling your lungs with air, and exhaling slowly through your mouth. Repeat this pattern for several minutes to promote relaxation and oxygenation.

3. **Yoga:** Engage in a gentle yoga practice that focuses on stretching, movement, and breath awareness. Flow through a series of yoga poses, paying attention to the sensations in your body and the rhythm of your breath. Choose poses that promote detoxification, such as twists, forward bends, and inversions, to stimulate circulation and release toxins from the body.

4. **Nature Walk:** Spend time in nature, connecting with the natural world and grounding yourself in the present moment. Take a leisurely walk in the park, forest, or beach, and immerse yourself in the sights, sounds, and sensations of the outdoors. Allow nature to nourish your senses and soothe your soul.

5. **Journaling:** Set aside time for reflective journaling, allowing yourself to explore your thoughts, feelings, and experiences. Write freely about your detox journey, expressing gratitude for the progress you've made and releasing any emotions or concerns that arise. Use journal prompts to deepen your self-awareness and gain insights into your inner world.

6. **Creative Expression:** Engage in creative activities that promote self-expression and emotional release. Experiment with painting, drawing, writing, or crafting as a means of processing and expressing your thoughts and emotions. Allow your creativity to flow freely without judgment or expectation.

7. **Self-Care Rituals:** Treat yourself to nourishing self-care rituals that promote relaxation and rejuvenation. Take a warm bath with Epsom salts and essential oils, indulge in a soothing cup of herbal tea, or pamper yourself with a gentle massage or self-massage using aromatic oils.

Creating Your Day 6 Mind-Body Detox Routine

Here's how you can create a personalized mind-body detox routine for Day 6:

1. **Morning Meditation:** Start your day with a guided meditation focused on relaxation, gratitude, and intention setting for the day ahead.

2. **Deep Breathing Breaks:** Take several breaks throughout the day to practice deep breathing exercises, pausing to center yourself and release tension.

3. **Yoga Practice:** Dedicate time to a gentle yoga practice that includes detoxifying poses and mindful movement. Focus on linking breath with movement and cultivating a sense of inner peace and balance.

4. **Nature Connection:** Spend time outdoors, connecting with nature and grounding yourself in the present moment. Take a mindful walk, breathe in the fresh air, and appreciate the beauty of the natural world around you.

5. **Journaling Session:** Set aside time for reflective journaling, exploring your thoughts, emotions, and insights gained from your detox journey. Write freely and authentically, allowing your words to flow without censorship.

6. **Creative Expression:** Engage in a creative activity that speaks to your soul, whether it's painting, writing poetry, or playing

music. Allow your creativity to be a source of inspiration, healing, and self-discovery.

7. **Evening Self-Care Ritual:** Wind down in the evening with a self-care ritual that nourishes your body, mind, and spirit. Treat yourself to a warm bath, indulge in a cup of herbal tea, and practice relaxation techniques before bedtime.

Conclusion

Day 6 of your detox journey is an opportunity to incorporate mind-body practices that support detoxification and stress reduction. By dedicating time to meditation, deep breathing, yoga, nature connection, journaling, creative expression, and self-care rituals, you'll nourish your mind, body, and spirit and enhance the benefits of your detox regimen. Cultivate a sense of inner peace, balance, and well-being as you continue on your journey toward greater health and vitality. Cheers to a day of mind-body nourishment and transformation on your detox journey!

CHAPTER TEN

Day 7: Reflecting on Your Detox Week and Creating a Post-Detox Plan

Congratulations on reaching Day 7 of your detox journey! As you near the end of your detox week, it's essential to take time for reflection, gratitude, and planning for the future. Day 7 is an opportunity to reflect on your experiences, celebrate your achievements, and create a post-detox plan that will support your ongoing health and well-being. By taking stock of what you've learned and setting intentions for the future, you can continue to build on the progress you've made during your detox and maintain a healthy lifestyle moving forward.

Reflecting on Your Detox Week

Take some time to reflect on your experiences and insights gained during your detox week. Consider the following questions:

1. **What were the highlights of your detox journey?**
2. **What challenges did you encounter, and how did you overcome them?**
3. **How did your body feel throughout the week?**
4. **What changes did you notice in your energy levels, mood, and overall well-being?**

5. **What did you learn about your habits, cravings, and relationship with food?**

6. **Did you discover any new foods, recipes, or practices that you enjoyed?**

7. **What insights did you gain about your mind-body connection and self-care needs?**

8. **What are you grateful for as you reflect on your detox experience?**

Take time to journal about your reflections, allowing yourself to express gratitude for the journey you've been on and acknowledging the growth and transformation you've experienced.

Creating a Post-Detox Plan

As you transition out of your detox week, it's important to create a post-detox plan that will support your ongoing health and well-being. Consider the following elements when designing your plan:

1. **Nutrition:** Continue to prioritize whole, nutrient-dense foods in your diet, including plenty of fruits, vegetables, whole grains, lean proteins, and healthy fats. Aim to maintain a balanced and varied diet that nourishes your body and supports your energy levels and overall health.

2. **Hydration:** Stay hydrated by drinking plenty of water throughout the day. Aim to drink at least eight glasses of water daily, and consider incorporating hydrating beverages such as herbal teas, infused water, and coconut water into your routine.

3. **Physical Activity:** Continue to incorporate regular physical activity into your daily routine to support your overall health and well-being. Choose activities that you enjoy, whether it's walking, cycling, yoga, or dancing, and aim for at least 30 minutes of moderate exercise most days of the week.

4. **Mind-Body Practices:** Maintain a regular practice of mind-body techniques such as meditation, deep breathing, yoga, and mindfulness to support stress reduction, relaxation, and emotional well-being. Schedule time for these practices each day to cultivate a sense of balance and inner peace.

5. **Sleep:** Prioritize restful sleep by establishing a consistent sleep schedule and creating a relaxing bedtime routine. Aim for 7-9 hours of quality sleep each night, and create a sleep environment that is conducive to rest and relaxation.

6. **Self-Care:** Continue to prioritize self-care practices that nourish your body, mind, and spirit. Make time for activities that bring you joy, relaxation, and fulfillment, whether it's spending time in nature, indulging in a hobby, or connecting with loved ones.

7. **Reflection and Planning:** Schedule regular check-ins with yourself to reflect on your progress, set intentions, and adjust your goals as needed. Use journaling, meditation, or visualization techniques to clarify your vision for your health and well-being and create actionable steps to achieve your goals.

Sample Post-Detox Plan

Here's an example of a post-detox plan that incorporates the elements mentioned above:

- **Nutrition:** Continue to prioritize whole foods, including plenty of fruits, vegetables, whole grains, lean proteins, and healthy fats. Incorporate detox-friendly meals and recipes into your regular diet and experiment with new flavors and ingredients.

- **Hydration:** Drink at least eight glasses of water daily and incorporate hydrating beverages such as herbal teas, infused water, and coconut water into your routine.

- **Physical Activity:** Engage in regular physical activity, including a mix of cardiovascular exercise, strength training, and flexibility exercises. Schedule workouts that you enjoy and make movement a priority in your daily life.

- **Mind-Body Practices:** Dedicate time each day to mind-body practices such as meditation, deep breathing, yoga, and mindfulness. Practice techniques that promote relaxation, stress reduction, and emotional well-being.

- **Sleep:** Prioritize restful sleep by establishing a consistent sleep schedule, creating a relaxing bedtime routine, and optimizing your sleep environment for comfort and tranquility.

- **Self-Care:** Make self-care a priority by scheduling regular activities that nourish your body, mind, and spirit. Treat yourself to massages, baths, nature walks, or creative pursuits that bring you joy and relaxation.

- **Reflection and Planning:** Schedule regular check-ins with yourself to reflect on your progress, set intentions, and adjust your goals as needed. Use journaling, meditation, or visualization techniques to clarify your vision for your health and well-being and create actionable steps to achieve your goals.

Conclusion

Day 7 of your detox journey is a time for reflection, celebration, and planning for the future. Take time to acknowledge and appreciate the progress you've made during your detox week, and use your reflections to create a post-detox plan that will support your ongoing health and well-being. By prioritizing nutrition, hydration, physical activity, mind-body practices, sleep, self-care, and reflection, you can continue to cultivate a lifestyle that promotes vitality, balance, and resilience. Cheers to your journey toward optimal health and well-being!

BONUS

SOME HOLISTIC APPROACHES TO KNOW

Juice Fasting:

Definition: Juice fasting, also known as juice cleansing or juice detoxification, involves consuming only fruit and vegetable juices for a specified period while abstaining from solid foods. It's often done as a short-term dietary cleanse or detox to eliminate toxins, promote weight loss, and improve overall health.

Ingredients: Juice fasting requires fresh fruits and vegetables, preferably organic, and a juicer or blender to extract the juice. Common ingredients used in juice fasting include leafy greens, carrots, celery, cucumbers, apples, beets, ginger, and citrus fruits.

How to Prepare: Preparing for a juice fast involves selecting a variety of fruits and vegetables, washing them thoroughly, and juicing them to extract the liquid. It's important to drink freshly prepared juices immediately to retain their nutritional value and minimize exposure to air and light, which can degrade certain nutrients.

Dosage: The duration of a juice fast can vary depending on individual goals and preferences. Some people may choose to fast for a few days, while others may extend the fast for a week or longer. It's essential to listen to your body's cues and break the fast if you experience significant discomfort or adverse effects.

How to Use: During a juice fast, participants typically consume freshly prepared fruit and vegetable juices throughout the day, drinking them at regular intervals to maintain hydration and energy levels. It's important to drink plenty of water in addition to juice to prevent dehydration and support detoxification processes.

Side Effects: While juice fasting may offer potential health benefits such as weight loss, improved digestion, and increased energy levels, it can also pose risks, especially if done for an extended period or without proper guidance. Potential side effects of juice fasting may include nutrient deficiencies, blood sugar fluctuations, dizziness, fatigue, headaches, and gastrointestinal upset. Juice fasting may not be suitable for everyone, especially those with certain medical conditions such as diabetes, kidney disease, or eating disorders. It's important to consult with a healthcare provider or registered dietitian before starting a juice fast, especially if you have underlying health concerns or are taking medications. Additionally, it's advisable to transition gradually into and out of a juice fast to minimize digestive discomfort and support long-term dietary changes.

Lemon Water:

Definition: Lemon water is a beverage made by squeezing fresh lemon juice into water. It's commonly consumed for its refreshing taste and potential health benefits.

Ingredients: Lemon water requires fresh lemon juice and water. Some people may also add additional ingredients such as honey, mint, or ginger for flavor enhancement.

How to Prepare: Preparing lemon water involves squeezing the juice of one or more fresh lemons into a glass of water and stirring to combine. The ratio of lemon juice to water can be adjusted according to personal taste preferences.

Dosage: There isn't a specific dosage for lemon water, but incorporating it into your daily routine can provide potential health benefits. Aim to drink one or more glasses of lemon water per day, preferably on an empty stomach in the morning or throughout the day for hydration and refreshment.

How to Use: Lemon water can be enjoyed cold, at room temperature, or warm, depending on personal preference. It can be consumed as a standalone beverage or incorporated into other drinks such as teas or smoothies. Some people also use lemon water as a flavor enhancer for cooking or salad dressings.

Side Effects: Lemon water is generally well-tolerated by most people when consumed in moderation. However, some individuals may experience side effects such as heartburn, acid reflux, or tooth erosion due to the acidic nature of lemon juice. It's important to rinse your mouth with plain water after drinking lemon water and avoid brushing your teeth immediately to protect tooth enamel. If you have specific health concerns or dietary restrictions, consult with a healthcare provider or registered dietitian before making significant changes to your diet.

Lymphatic Drainage Massage:

Definition: Lymphatic drainage massage is a specialized massage technique designed to stimulate the lymphatic system and encourage the natural flow of lymph fluid throughout the body. It's often used to reduce swelling, promote detoxification, boost immunity, and support overall health and well-being.

Ingredients: Lymphatic drainage massage requires no specific ingredients, as it involves manual manipulation of the skin and underlying tissues to stimulate lymphatic circulation. However, some therapists may use a gentle massage oil or lotion to reduce friction and enhance the massage experience.

How to Prepare: Preparing for a lymphatic drainage massage involves selecting a qualified massage therapist trained in lymphatic drainage techniques and scheduling a session. It's important to communicate any health concerns or preferences with the therapist before the massage begins.

Dosage: The frequency and duration of lymphatic drainage massage sessions can vary depending on individual needs and goals. Some people may benefit from regular sessions to address specific health issues, while others may use lymphatic drainage massage occasionally for relaxation or maintenance.

How to Use: During a lymphatic drainage massage, the therapist uses gentle, rhythmic movements to stimulate lymphatic circulation and encourage the removal of toxins and waste products from the body. The massage may focus on specific areas of the body, such as the arms, legs, abdomen, or face, depending on individual needs and concerns.

Side Effects: Lymphatic drainage massage is generally safe for most people when performed by a qualified therapist. However, some individuals may experience mild side effects such as temporary soreness, fatigue, or increased urination following a massage session. These side effects are usually temporary and subside with time. If you have specific health conditions such as cancer, lymphedema, or circulatory disorders, or if you're pregnant, it's essential to consult with a healthcare provider before undergoing lymphatic drainage massage to ensure it's safe and appropriate for you.

Milk Thistle Supplements:

Definition: Milk thistle supplements are dietary supplements made from the seeds of the milk thistle plant (Silybum marianum). They are known for their potential liver-supportive properties and are commonly used to promote liver health and detoxification.

Ingredients: Milk thistle supplements typically contain extracts from the seeds of the milk thistle plant, standardized to contain a specific amount of the active compound silymarin. Other ingredients may include fillers, binders, and additional herbs or botanicals.

How to Prepare: Preparing for milk thistle supplement use involves selecting a reputable product from a trusted manufacturer and following the recommended dosage instructions provided on the product packaging or as advised by a healthcare provider.

Dosage: The recommended dosage of milk thistle supplements can vary depending on the specific formulation and individual needs. It's essential to follow the dosage instructions carefully and not exceed the recommended dose without consulting with a healthcare provider.

How to Use: Milk thistle supplements are typically taken orally with water or another beverage, preferably with meals to enhance absorption and minimize gastrointestinal upset. Some supplements may recommend a specific dosing schedule or additional dietary and lifestyle recommendations to support liver health and detoxification.

Side Effects: Milk thistle supplements are generally well-tolerated by most people when used as directed, but some individuals may experience side effects such as gastrointestinal upset, allergic reactions, or interactions with medications. It's essential to read the ingredient list carefully and avoid supplements containing ingredients that may trigger allergic reactions or interact with medications you're taking. Pregnant or breastfeeding women, individuals with certain medical conditions, or those taking medications should consult with a healthcare provider before using milk thistle supplements. Additionally, it's important to choose supplements from reputable brands with third-party testing and certifications to ensure product quality and purity.

Oil Pulling:

Definition: Oil pulling is an ancient Ayurvedic practice that involves swishing oil around in the mouth for a specified period, typically 10 to 20 minutes, to promote oral health and detoxification.

Ingredients: Oil pulling requires a natural oil such as coconut oil, sesame oil, or sunflower oil. These oils are believed to have antimicrobial properties and may help remove bacteria, plaque, and toxins from the mouth.

How to Prepare: Preparing for oil pulling involves selecting a suitable oil and ensuring that it's in liquid form, preferably at room temperature. Some people may choose to add a few drops of essential oil, such as peppermint or tea tree oil, for flavor or additional benefits.

Dosage: The recommended duration for oil pulling is typically 10 to 20 minutes, although some people may choose to swish the oil for longer periods. It's important to start with a shorter duration, such as 5 minutes, and gradually increase the time as you become accustomed to the practice.

How to Use: To perform oil pulling, take a tablespoon of oil and swish it around in your mouth, making sure to pull it through your teeth and around your gums. Avoid swallowing the oil, as it may contain bacteria and toxins removed from the mouth. After the designated time, spit out the oil into a trash bin and rinse your mouth thoroughly with water.

Side Effects: Oil pulling is generally safe for most people when done correctly, but some individuals may experience side effects such as nausea, upset stomach, or a gag reflex when swishing the oil. These side effects are typically mild and temporary and may subside with continued practice. If you experience any discomfort or adverse reactions, discontinue oil pulling and consult with a healthcare provider. Additionally, oil pulling is not a substitute for regular oral hygiene practices such as brushing and flossing, so it's important to continue these habits for optimal oral health.

Oxygen Therapy:

Definition: Oxygen therapy is a medical treatment that involves administering supplemental oxygen to individuals with breathing difficulties or low blood oxygen levels. It's used to improve oxygen delivery to tissues and organs, relieve symptoms of hypoxemia (low blood oxygen), and support respiratory function.

Ingredients: Oxygen therapy typically requires medical-grade oxygen, which is administered using various delivery systems such as nasal cannulas, oxygen masks, or oxygen concentrators. The oxygen itself is the active ingredient in this therapy.

How to Prepare: Preparing for oxygen therapy involves assessing the individual's oxygen needs, determining the appropriate flow rate and delivery system, and ensuring access to medical-grade oxygen and necessary equipment.

Dosage: The dosage of oxygen therapy is prescribed by a healthcare provider based on factors such as the severity of hypoxemia, underlying health conditions, and individual oxygen requirements. Oxygen flow rates are measured in liters per minute (LPM), and the prescribed flow rate may vary depending on the specific situation.

How to Use: Oxygen therapy is typically administered under the guidance of healthcare professionals, either in a hospital setting, outpatient clinic, or at home. The delivery system and flow rate are adjusted as needed to maintain adequate blood oxygen levels and relieve symptoms of hypoxemia.

Side Effects: While oxygen therapy is generally safe and well-tolerated when used as prescribed, excessive oxygen supplementation can lead to complications such as oxygen toxicity, respiratory depression, and absorption atelectasis (collapse of lung tissue). It's essential to follow the prescribed oxygen flow rate and usage instructions carefully and to monitor for signs of oxygen toxicity or respiratory distress. Individuals with certain respiratory conditions such as chronic obstructive pulmonary disease (COPD) may require careful monitoring and adjustment of oxygen therapy to prevent complications.

Probiotic Supplements:

Definition: Probiotic supplements are dietary supplements containing live bacteria or yeasts that are believed to provide health benefits by restoring or maintaining a healthy balance of gut microbiota (the community of microorganisms in the digestive tract).

Ingredients: Probiotic supplements contain various strains of beneficial bacteria or yeasts, such as Lactobacillus, Bifidobacterium, Saccharomyces, or Streptococcus. These microorganisms are typically present in fermented foods like yogurt, kefir, sauerkraut, and kimchi.

How to Prepare: Preparing for probiotic supplement use involves selecting a suitable product from a reputable manufacturer and following the recommended dosage instructions provided on the product packaging or as advised by a healthcare provider.

Dosage: The recommended dosage of probiotic supplements can vary depending on the specific formulation, strain, and individual needs. It's essential to follow the dosage instructions carefully and to choose a supplement with strains and doses supported by scientific evidence for the intended health benefits.

How to Use: Probiotic supplements are typically taken orally with water or another beverage, preferably with meals to enhance absorption and minimize gastrointestinal upset. Some supplements may recommend refrigeration to maintain the viability of live probiotic cultures.

Side Effects: Probiotic supplements are generally safe for most people when used as directed, but some individuals may experience side effects such as bloating, gas, diarrhea, or abdominal discomfort, especially when first starting probiotic supplementation or with high doses. These side effects are usually mild and temporary and may subside with continued use. It's important to choose probiotic supplements from reputable brands with third-party testing and certifications to ensure product quality and potency. Individuals with certain medical conditions, compromised immune systems, or allergies to specific probiotic strains should consult with a healthcare provider before using probiotic supplements. Additionally, probiotic supplements are not a substitute for a balanced diet and healthy lifestyle, so it's essential to focus on overall dietary patterns and gut health practices for optimal well-being.

Raw Food Diet:

Definition: A raw food diet is a dietary approach that emphasizes consuming uncooked, unprocessed, and predominantly plant-based foods. It's based on the belief that cooking destroys enzymes, vitamins, and other nutrients in food and that consuming raw foods can promote better health and vitality.

Ingredients: A raw food diet includes a variety of fruits, vegetables, nuts, seeds, sprouted grains, legumes, and seaweed. Common raw food staples include salads, smoothies, raw fruits and vegetables, nuts and seeds, raw dairy products (such as unpasteurized milk and cheese), and fermented foods (such as sauerkraut and kimchi).

How to Prepare: Preparing for a raw food diet involves selecting fresh, organic, and preferably locally sourced ingredients. Food is typically eaten raw or minimally processed, such as juicing, blending, soaking, sprouting, or dehydrating at low temperatures to preserve nutrients.

Dosage: There isn't a specific dosage for a raw food diet, as it depends on individual preferences, nutritional needs, and health goals. Some people may choose to follow a fully raw diet, while others may incorporate raw foods into their diet alongside cooked foods.

How to Use: On a raw food diet, food is consumed in its natural state, with minimal processing or cooking. This may include eating raw fruits and vegetables, salads, smoothies, raw nuts and seeds, and raw dairy products. It's important to practice food safety and hygiene when handling raw foods to prevent contamination and foodborne illness.

Side Effects: While a raw food diet can provide numerous health benefits such as increased consumption of vitamins, minerals, fiber, and antioxidants, it can also pose risks if not balanced properly. Potential side effects of a raw food diet may include nutrient deficiencies (such as vitamin B12, iron, calcium, and protein), digestive issues (such as bloating, gas, and diarrhea), and foodborne illness from consuming raw or undercooked foods. It's essential to plan meals carefully to ensure adequate nutrient intake and to listen to your body's cues to prevent deficiencies or imbalances. Individuals with certain health conditions, such as gastrointestinal disorders or compromised immune systems, should consult with a healthcare provider or registered dietitian before starting a raw food diet.

Sauna Therapy:

Definition: Sauna therapy involves exposing the body to high temperatures in a sauna or sweat lodge to induce sweating and promote relaxation, detoxification, and overall well-being. It's used in various cultures around the world for its therapeutic effects on the body and mind.

Ingredients: Sauna therapy requires a sauna or sweat lodge, typically heated to temperatures ranging from 150°F to 195°F (65°C to 90°C). Some saunas use dry heat (such as Finnish saunas), while others use moist heat (such as steam rooms or Turkish baths). Water for hydration is essential during sauna sessions to prevent dehydration.

How to Prepare: Preparing for sauna therapy involves selecting a suitable sauna or sweat lodge and ensuring that it's properly heated to the desired temperature. It's important to hydrate adequately before, during, and after sauna sessions and to listen to your body's cues to prevent overheating.

Dosage: The duration and frequency of sauna therapy sessions can vary depending on individual preferences, tolerance to heat, and health goals. Some people may benefit from short, frequent sauna sessions, while others may prefer longer sessions less frequently.

How to Use: During a sauna session, individuals sit or lie comfortably in the sauna, allowing the body to heat up and sweat. It's essential to stay hydrated by drinking water or electrolyte-rich beverages and to listen to your body's signals to prevent overheating or dehydration. After the sauna session, it's advisable to cool down gradually and rehydrate to replenish lost fluids.

Side Effects: Sauna therapy is generally safe for most people when used appropriately, but it can pose risks if not practiced correctly. Potential side effects of sauna therapy may include dehydration, heat exhaustion, heatstroke, dizziness, fainting, and exacerbation of certain medical conditions (such as cardiovascular disease or low blood pressure). It's important to stay hydrated, limit sauna sessions to a safe duration (typically 15 to 20 minutes), and avoid excessive heat exposure if pregnant, breastfeeding, or if you have certain health conditions. Individuals with underlying health concerns should consult with a healthcare provider before starting sauna therapy to ensure it's safe and appropriate for them.

Seaweed Wraps:

Definition: Seaweed wraps, also known as seaweed body wraps or seaweed body masks, are spa treatments that involve applying a mixture of seaweed-based products to the body and wrapping it in plastic or cloth. They are believed to help detoxify the skin, improve circulation, and promote relaxation.

Ingredients: Seaweed wraps typically contain various types of seaweed extracts, such as bladderwrack, kelp, or laminaria, which are rich in vitamins, minerals, antioxidants, and other beneficial compounds. Additional ingredients may include clay, essential oils, herbal extracts, and moisturizing agents.

How to Prepare: Preparing for a seaweed wrap involves selecting a suitable seaweed-based product or mixture, such as a pre-made seaweed wrap solution or a DIY blend using powdered seaweed and other ingredients. The skin is typically exfoliated and cleansed before the seaweed mixture is applied.

Dosage: The duration of a seaweed wrap treatment can vary depending on individual preferences and spa protocols. A typical seaweed wrap session may last 30 to 60 minutes, during which the body is wrapped in seaweed-soaked bandages or plastic wrap to enhance absorption and maximize the benefits of the treatment.

How to Use: During a seaweed wrap treatment, the seaweed mixture is applied to the skin and massaged or brushed onto the body, focusing on areas of concern such as cellulite or dry skin. The body is then wrapped in plastic or cloth to promote heat retention and allow the seaweed to penetrate the skin. After the designated time, the wrap is removed, and the skin may be rinsed or moisturized as desired.

Side Effects: Seaweed wraps are generally considered safe for most people when performed by trained professionals or used according to package instructions. However, some individuals may experience skin irritation, allergic reactions, or sensitivity to certain ingredients in the seaweed mixture. It's essential to perform a patch test before using seaweed wraps extensively and to consult with a healthcare provider if you have underlying skin conditions or allergies. Additionally, pregnant or breastfeeding women and individuals with certain medical conditions should consult with a healthcare provider before undergoing seaweed wrap treatments.

Skin Detox Masks:

Definition: Skin detox masks, also known as detoxifying facial masks or purifying face masks, are skincare products designed to remove impurities, excess oil, and toxins from the skin, leaving it feeling clean, refreshed, and revitalized.

Ingredients: Skin detox masks may contain a variety of ingredients chosen for their detoxifying, purifying, and clarifying properties. Common ingredients include clay (such as kaolin or bentonite), charcoal, activated charcoal, mud, seaweed, herbal extracts, antioxidants, and essential oils.

How to Prepare: Preparing for a skin detox mask involves selecting a suitable product based on skin type and concerns. Some masks come in pre-packaged single-use packets or jars, while others may be mixed with water or another liquid to form a paste before application.

Dosage: The frequency of skin detox mask application can vary depending on individual skin needs and preferences. Some people may use a detox mask once or twice a week as part of their skincare routine, while others may use them less frequently or as needed.

How to Use: To use a skin detox mask, apply a thin, even layer to clean, dry skin, avoiding the eye area and lips. Allow the mask to dry completely, typically for 10 to 20 minutes, before rinsing it off with warm water. Follow up with a moisturizer or other skincare products as needed.

Side Effects: Skin detox masks are generally safe for most people when used as directed, but some individuals may experience skin irritation, redness, or dryness, especially if they have sensitive skin or allergies to certain ingredients. It's essential to perform a patch test before using a new detox mask and to discontinue use if any adverse reactions occur. Additionally, overuse of detox masks or leaving them on for too long can lead to excessive dryness or irritation, so it's important to follow package instructions and listen to your skin's needs. If you have specific skin concerns or medical conditions, consult with a dermatologist or skincare professional before incorporating detox masks into your skincare routine.

Sleep:

Definition: Sleep is a natural, recurring state of rest characterized by reduced consciousness, decreased sensory activity, and inhibited voluntary muscle movement. It's essential for overall health and well-being, playing a crucial role in physical and mental restoration, memory consolidation, and immune function.

Ingredients: Sleep requires no specific ingredients but is influenced by various factors such as environmental conditions, lifestyle habits, and individual health factors. Creating a conducive sleep environment and practicing good sleep hygiene can help promote quality sleep.

How to Prepare: Preparing for sleep involves establishing a regular sleep schedule, creating a relaxing bedtime routine, and optimizing your sleep environment. This may include dimming the lights, reducing screen time before bed, avoiding caffeine and heavy meals close to bedtime, and creating a comfortable sleep environment with a supportive mattress and pillows.

Dosage: The recommended amount of sleep varies depending on age, with adults typically needing 7-9 hours of sleep per night for optimal health and functioning. It's essential to prioritize quality sleep and aim for sufficient duration to feel rested and refreshed upon waking.

How to Use: To promote better sleep, establish a consistent sleep-wake schedule by going to bed and waking up at the same time each day, even on weekends. Create a relaxing bedtime routine to signal to your body that it's time to wind down, such as reading, taking a warm bath, or practicing relaxation techniques like deep breathing or meditation. Ensure your sleep environment is conducive to sleep by keeping the room cool, dark, and quiet.

Side Effects: Chronic sleep deprivation or poor sleep quality can lead to various adverse effects on physical and mental health, including fatigue, irritability, impaired cognitive function, weakened immune system, increased risk of chronic diseases such as obesity, diabetes, and cardiovascular disease, and mood disorders such as depression and anxiety. It's essential to prioritize sleep as part of a healthy lifestyle and seek professional help if you experience persistent sleep problems or symptoms of sleep disorders.

THE END

www.ingramcontent.com/pod-product-compliance
Lightning Source LLC
Chambersburg PA
CBHW082354220526
45470CB00008B/2739